Fifth Dimensional Healing

Crystal Wizdom and the Five Elements of Multidimensional Healing

Wayne "Lone Eagle" Darling

Words of Wizdom International, Inc.

ISBN: 1-884695-11-6
Fifth Dimensional Healing

Cover and Interior Design: Marilyn Hager

Words of Wizdom International, Inc.,
Orders Toll Free in USA: 1-800-834-7612
Website: www.wizdombooks.com
Email: info@wizdombooks.com

Printed in Canada
First Printing: January 1999

1 3 5 7 9 2 4 6 8

Dedication

I dedicate this book to my Spiritual Guides and
all the Beings who have helped
and guided me on my journey.

For Red Feather, Long Feather, Crystal,
Many Lives, Julian Patrick O'Reilly
and all the rest of you,
with all my Love.

And for you,
Sam,
my four-legged best friend.

Love and Thanks to my Publisher,
Tracy O'Reilly.

Table of Contents

Introduction. xi

Part I: The Five Elements in Healing. 3

Fifth Dimensional Healing Elements 8

The Element of Air
Celestial Constellations. 11
Constellations 13
Planets 14
Sacred Smoke & Incense. 15
Aromatherapy 16
Feathers 17

The Element of Earth
Vortex Energies & Ley Lines. 21
Stonehenge & Avebury, England 22
The Great Pyramid of Giza, Egypt. 22
Uluru & Katatjara, Australia 23
Newgrange, Ireland 23
The Four Corners, USA. 24
Mt. Shasta, USA. 24
Garden of the Gods, USA 25
Herbs, Healing Plants & Homeopathy 26
Crystals & Minerals. 27

The Element of Water
Healing Waters, Sacred Springs & Wells. 31
Chalice Well, England. 31
The Healing Hole, North Bimini, Bahamas. . . 32
Australian Waterholes. 34

Katherine Gorge, Australia. 35
Abalone 35
Elixirs 36

The Element of Fire
Solar & Volcanic Energies 41
Kundalini 42
Candles. 43

The Element of Ether: Sacred Synthesis
The Element of Ether. 47
Synthesis 48
Love 49

Part II: The Crystal People
Cleansing Your Crystal 53
Crystal Enlightenment Through
Crystal & Mineral Healing 54
Alexandrite 55
Amethyst Phantom 56
Angelite 57
Apophyllite & Ulexite. 58
Azurite 59
Bloodstone & Sugilite 60
Candle Quartz 61
Chrysocolla 62
Cinnabar, Malachite & Citrine 63
Citrine & Amber 64
Crystal Quartz Clusters & Black Tourmaline . 65
Dioptase & Moldavite. 66
Galena. 67
Green Garnet & Sugilite 69
Herkimer Diamonds & Apophyllite 70

Kunzite. 71
Lepidolite & Tourmaline. 73
Malachite & Aventurine 74
Moldavite. 75
Moldavite & Ulexite 77
Obsidian. 78
Purple Fluorite. 79
Rhodochrosite 80
Strawberry Quartz rutilated with Lepidolite . 81
Sugilite, Moldavite & Ulexite 82
Sugilite, Purple Fluorite & Blue Kyanite 83

Power Packs 85

Crystal Meditation Wheel 87

Copper Pyramids 89

About the Author 91
About the Publisher 93

Introduction

This title might lead some to expect a large, technical and somewhat complicated book. In fact, as we evolve, we can allow things to become simple once again.

This is not a complete guide to anything, but merely provides basic, essential knowledge with which every healer can proceed into multidimensional healing. Only you will know how to make this knowledge complete and how it can work for and with you.

The clue to using this book effectively is to blend and combine all five elements of healing instead of choosing one or two. When all five are used together, the value is greater than the sum of the parts.

I am not a physician and all information shared by me in this book is based on my present and past life knowledge, as well as my experiences. None of this information is meant to take the place of a doctor's supervision where illness is concerned.

Many American states and foreign countries now recognize some forms of alternative healing and we can look forward to more of this as time goes by.

Always remember, whatever you do, do it with love in your heart and surround yourself with white light. A healthy mind is a healthy spirit which is a healthy person. This brings beautiful self-esteem. We are the masters of our own destinies, and we are our thoughts, so keep them positive. And always say to yourself, I AM. I am love, I am light, I am the universe, because I AM.

I always say to my friends, "When you sleep with crystals you'll wake up stoned". And when I wake up in the mornings after sleeping with 5 crystal balls, over 600 lbs. of quartz crystals and points and many other minerals in my bedroom, I return from crystal journeys in the dreamstate. What a wonderful and beautiful feeling to be surrounded by them.

Crystals and minerals are Mother Nature's way of greeting us, and sending us love from our Earth Mother and from our Creator. I always call them my Crystal People, for they have personalities and characteristics just like we do.

Crystals are known to be thought transmittors and senders, but what few people know is that crystals are love. To work successfully with a crystal, you must first give it love, and enter into a love vibration. When your heart chakra opens and you can feel waves of love being released, you can attune with your crystal to manifest the highest level of healing and interaction.

I've experimented with many people, as well as my own personal experiments. We all ask our crystals for healing, guidance, manifestation, awareness, heightened intuition, etc. But if you really want to connect with your crystal on a very deep level, turn on some beautiful music that speaks to your soul, grab your crystal, hug it, hold it, talk to it, and dance with it. After a while, you'll notice a subtle change; you are no longer leading the dance . . . the crystal is!

This is not only a way to bond with your crystal, it is a deep and moving healing. I've seen so many people break down and cry as they start releasing unknown emotional wounds. Something about the combination of the musical vibration which speaks to your essence, and the spiritual connection with your crystal can act as a catalyst to unblock emotions that were held back deep inside. If you get nothing else from these pages, learn to love your crystal and dance with it, because you are it's keeper, and it is your friend.

If your inner child is wounded, which is the case in many people where it is carried over from childhood, dancing with your crystal will be a great way to allow your inner child to surface, and to talk to him or her. There are many great books available on how to heal your inner child; this approach is instinctive instead of mental. The movement of sacred dance helps release trapped patterns and emotions.

Also, if you find the idea of dancing with a crystal silly, or feel inhibited about doing it, let your inner child take over, since this part of you will be delighted to be allowed to play and enjoy this freedom of movement.

Fifth Dimensional Healing

Part I

The Five Elements in Healing

When our planet shifted from the third dimension to the fourth, linear thinking started to be cumbersome. We have begun to realize that a wholistic and holographic approach to life is the only way to wholeness and health, and that "going with the flow" is an easier way to operate than in a linear manner. So many healing tools have been provided for us that all we need to do is use them.

This is not a how-to manual. This book touches on how we can bring in the energies of these many "helpers" to enhance the outcome we seek, which is perfect health and happiness.

What is a fifth dimensional healer? First of all, it is a healer who sees things as already being in a state of perfection. The eyes are the greatest tools of the fifth dimensional healer. The two physical eyes and the third eye are used as a triangle of vision and, as lasers, are capable of creating the picture of perfection the healer visualizes. A fifth dimensional healer does not see the illusion of imperfection. In order to return something to a state of perfection, you must already *see* it as being perfect. This is perhaps one of the hardest things to do, since we so easily become wrapped up in the energy of "the moment."

For those of us who have difficulty believing

our eyes can make a change, focus on a small cloud with the intent to dissolve it, and continue until the cloud is gone. It will take a very short time to accomplish your goal, and you will be surprised and delighted at the power of your eyes and intent.

If you are looking into a mirror at your overweight body and saying silently to yourself, "I look terrible; I am fat and ugly," then you are perpetuating this situation and making it your reality.

Realize your thoughts are a powerful mantra or affirmation, and *what you focus on expands*. Instead of being critical, use your eyes consciously to beam love through the mirror back to yourself. See yourself as beautiful, and allow yourself to feel that you are in a state of perfection. Things will adjust gradually and normally and you will have retained a sense of love and harmony all the way through.

The importance of this highly effective exercise should not be underestimated. Patience is a virtue, and you shoud remember it took time to reach the state you are currently in. Give yourself a chance to heal instead of expecting overnight miracles and quick fixes. To *heal* is to *love*; to *love* is to *heal*. Heal thyself and Love thyself.

The aboriginal people of Australia, also known as the first people on that continent, have a long and rich history of interdimensional healings and connections with the star systems. In their secret teachings, which they have tried to keep to themselves, we know they believe in a similar concept to the one outlined in this book. According to James G. Cowan in his book, *The Aborigine Tradition*, the Aborigines call it 'the fifth essence,' and believe that everything within the four elements of physical matter, otherwise known as air, earth, water and fire, is embued with the spiritual essence of the fifth, which is the energy of creation found in all stars.

When I read this, I was thankful to the Creator to realize that my life's path has brought me to the same spiritual belief the Aborigines have embraced for thousands of years. I have spent time in Australia and had the honor of meeting an Aborigine medicine man at one of their most sacred sites, Uluru. I was welcomed into the heart of an Aborigine family and shared their wonderful hospitality. The Aborigine energy is very unique on this planet; these people have retained an innocence rarely found on planet Earth.

Fifth Dimensional Healing Elements

Air
- Celestial Constellations
- Sacred Smoke & Incense
- Aromatherapy
- Feathers

Earth
- Vortex Energies & Ley Lines
- Herbs, Healing Plants & Homeopathy
- Crystals & Minerals

Water
- Healing Waters, Sacred Springs & Wells
- Abalone
- Elixirs

Fire
- Solar & Volcanic Energies & Kundalini
- Candles

Ether
- Synthesis
- Love

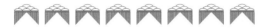

The
Element
of
AIR

Celestial Constellations

The heavenly bodies and constellations provide an unusual source of healing we seldom use. Most people are familiar with the basic attributes of their zodiac sign and those of their loved ones. We all know that Gemini is the communicator of the zodiac, Cancer is the family-oriented member, and Scorpio is the mysterious and secretive one.

Now take this information a step further. What if you are sadly lacking in communication skills? Has it ever occured to you that you can go out under the night sky, locate Gemini, and ask the being or energy field that is Gemini to assist you in improving your skills in this arena? In this way, if you do a little research on the meanings of planetary and constellation mythology, as well as simple astronomy, you will easily find the constellation which can assist in your empowerment.

Invite your spiritual guides and teachers to come in and inspire you in making these connections with the starry bodies and cosmic energies.

You cannot always see the constellation in the sky with which you may wish to connect, depending on the time of year and which hemisphere you are located in. If you cannot find what you need in the night sky, it is just as effective to use a book, photo or map outline of the constellations.

For instance, open a book to the constellation of the Southern Cross if you are in the northern hemisphere, and put it under your pillow. Ask the beings of the Southern Cross to come to you in dreamstate and assist you in becoming more focused, since the cross is an intersection point and therefore can help you with goal-oriented matters and targeting issues.

Always remember, we had to learn to crawl before we could walk, and as a healer we take one step at a time. Our guides will guide us and our spirits will enlighten us on the right path.

Below I provide a brief list of some of the main constellations and planets, so you can get familiar with them. If you enjoy this aspect of healing, I encourage you to investigate it more and would be happy if you write or e-mail me, sharing your experiences.

Constellations

ARIES	Impulsive, Fiery, Dynamic, Courageous, Self-starting
TAURUS	Stable, Sensual, Strong, Prosperous, Grounded
GEMINI	Communicative, Witty, Intellectual, Playful
CANCER	Nurturing, Loving, Family-oriented, Responsive
LEO	Charismatic, Leadership-oriented, Bold, Brave, Noble, Dramatic
VIRGO	Reliable, Industrious, Analytical, Precise, Healing
LIBRA	Balanced, Justice, Intellectual, Harmonious, Romantic, Fair-minded
SCORPIO	Passionate, Sexual, Penetrating, Powerful, Intense
SAGITTARIUS	Adventurous, Outgoing, Talkative, Optimistic
CAPRICORN	Pioneering, Persistent, Successful, Organized
AQUARIUS	Revolutionary, Visionary, Eccentric, Innovative, Futuristic
PISCES	Perceptive, Emotional, Cosmic, Psychic, Intuitive

ORION   Unconditional Love and Expansion

SIRIUS   Loyalty and Emotional Integration

PLEIADES   Time Travel and Advanced
                Civilizations

DELPHINUS   Emotional Balancing, Playfulness,
                Joy

Planets

VENUS   Love and Compassion

MERCURY   Intellect

MARS   Activity

MOON   Psychic and Emotional Realms

SUN   Physical Strength and Energy

NEPTUNE   Abundance and memories of
                Atlantis

SATURN   Knowledge, Learning, Karma

JUPITER   Abundance, Joy, Happiness

PLUTO   Sudden Change

URANUS   Astrological Assistance

If you find yourself unable to relate to your spouse and children, or unable to give or receive love, you would call on Venus and also the constellation of Cancer to assist you.

Are you having difficulty staying grounded and

achieving your earthly goals? Call on both Taurus and Capricorn as two well-grounded and focused constellations, and spend time in the wild, calling on Mother Earth herself.

If your problems are of a sexual nature, call on Scorpio, Venus and Jupiter to assist you with sexuality, love and happiness.

I could write many pages on this theme, but I only want to give you the clues and let you create your own reality. I'll leave it to you to work out which constellations and planets to call on, reminding you that the lists above are only the beginning. Remember that there are many less known constellations you can seek out with a good book or a very good astrologer. This research can be a lot of fun and open new doorways to you.

Sacred Smoke & Incense

Smoke created in a ceremonial ritual has been sacred to Native Americans and indigenous and aboriginal people of the world since time began.

Air is the element which carries the spiritual message of smoke to the Creator. A lot of importance is also placed on the symbolic shapes it adopts as it rises to the heavens and to the Creator. Learning to read the messages in smoke can be a very useful form of prophecy, especially if you ask Creator for a spiritual message.

Sacred smoke can be created by burning sage, pure tobacco, cedar, sweetgrass, and different herbs native to your area. Surround your space in white light, bless your space, and draw goodness and love into your heart. Sage in particular, known as Grandfather Sage, is a powerful plant growing wild in the western United States and has been honored for centuries by American Natives as being the ultimate cleanser and protector of spaces. It is said that no negative energies can withstand the intense cleansing aroma of Grandfather Sage. Whichever plant you choose, honor it before burning it.

If you are unable to obtain fresh or dried plants, even store-purchased incense can go a long way toward cleansing your space.

Aromatherapy

The vibrational and essential energy of the flower essences is carried to you via the element of air. This form of healing is light, airy and refreshing. A few drops of an essential oil like lavender or rose can permeate your room, or your bath water, and serves to change your mood to a much lighter one.

There are flower devas and fairy energies attached to these plant essences, so it would enhance and awaken your senses if you connect with these energies while delighting in a meditative state.

When purchasing aromatherapy oils, try to buy the purest and most natural ones available. The synthetic oils can provide the same general smell, but will not activate your energy field the same way as natural oils. Unfortunately, some of the best oils are more expensive than the synthetic ones, but less is more and you are better off with one or two bottles of high quality oil than a lot of inferior ones. The finest oils are the young living ones. If you can't locate them you can contact me for more information.

Feathers

The magic of feathers is that while they are of spirit, they are lighter than air and yet they can travel to the ground. Each time you come across a feather, see it as a spiritual message from one of your guides. Ask yourself what is on your mind at the time you see the feather. The feather is a sign that you are on the right path.

Feathers are excellent tools for energetic cleansing before a healing session. Use them as a fan with sage or sacred smoke to cleanse the energy field around the physical body. The feather carries away all that is negative and replaces it with a breath of fresh air.

Although it has become illegal to own eagle feathers and feathers of other birds of prey in the United States, American Natives have always used the feathers of these birds in their most sacred ceremonies, honoring Brother Eagle as being the highest on the spiritual ladder in the skies and closest to the Creator. In this manner, the spirit of Eagle, by way of his feathers, carries the messages, prayers, hopes and offerings of the people to the Creator, and a sacred bond is established.

While Eagle and Hawk feathers are like the Rolls Royces of the feather world, it is important to honor all feathers equally, and to remember that each feather is sacred, whether it is buzzard, chicken or crow.

So next time you see a feather while you are out walking, pick it up and thank the spirit of the bird who left it for you, and your spirit guide who placed it on your path. The more you recognize these signs, the easier it becomes for your guides and teachers to communicate with you. Your link to spirit becomes stronger and greater.

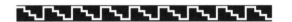

The
Element
of
EARTH

Vortex Energies
& Ley Lines

If we compare Mother Earth to our own bodies, her vortices are like our chakras and her ley lines are like our meridian system which acupuncturists use to stimulate energy flow. Earth is sprinkled with ley lines and vortices, which account for many mysteries we do not yet understand about our planet. The Bermuda Triangle in the Atlantic and The Dragon's Triangle in the Pacific are just two of these mysterious areas. Interdimensional travel can be accomplished at many power points on Mother Earth.

One of the most powerful ways to use the healing energies of Mother Earth is to find a strong vortex of energy, which is similar to a whirlwind of concentrated chi energy, and stand barefoot, sit or lie down on it. You will feel the power of your Earth Mother rising up to join with your energy to enhance it in whatever manner necessary.

We should take a leaf out of the books of the indigenous people of the planet, who all consider Mother Earth a living, breathing and conscious entity. They built their shrines, sacred sites and holy places on energy points, and many of them are found on intersection points where several ley lines cross.

There are famous vortices of many different types of energy, and I will list just a few below. However, you are just as likely to find an earth source of earth energy which is unknown but powerful right in your neighborhood.

Stonehenge & Avebury, England

While Avebury is known as an ancient fertility center where women celebrated sacred mysteries, Stonehenge has a penetrating and intense energy which is absolutely masculine. While the origins of Stonehenge are still steeped in mystery, it is my belief that apart from being a very important intersection point it is also an ancient communication "satellite" of sorts, where people communed with other beings in distant star systems. My intuitive feeling is that some day we will find Stonehenge is of Atlantean origin.

The Great Pyramid of Giza, Egypt

This man-made structure is built to precise mathematical ratio of PHI, according to Dr. G. Patrick Flanagan in his book, *Pyramid Power*. There is no other pyramid like it in the world, and it is aligned perpendicular to True North with an error of only 4'32" of one degree. Not only this, but the Great Pyramid is situated exactly on the 31 degree 9 minute meridian east of Greenwich, and on the 29 degree 58 minute 51 second North Latitude, which is an extremely siginificant location in that these meridians, if extended exactly, divided the land masses of earth into equal areas. The power of this vortex is enormous. While there are many books about the Egyptian pyramids, I highly recommend Dr. Flanagan's book as one of the best.

Uluru and Katatjara, Australia

These are two of the most sacred sites to Australian Aborigines. Uluru is considered the navel of their world, and is full of sacred sites for both men and women. It is a giant sandstone megalith, and is steeped in myth and legend. I feel, based on my own experiences there, that this is an interdimensional gateway.

Katatjara, which means "many heads," is sacred to women and men don't go there.

Newgrange, Ireland

Ireland is riddled with sacred sites, many interconnected on ley lines. Many of the true origins have been lost since Christianity arrived, wiping out the old ways. Newgrange is one of our planet's most important megalithic tombs, located on Irelands major ley line. The exterior is made of white quartz, and it is believed to have been built to align with the sun/moon at the time of the winter solstice, although some speculate it was originally aligned with the summer solstice, and that the earth meanwhile flipped its axis. Scientists are still puzzled by many mysterious features found here. It is a magnetic point and a place of great earth energy. There is a specific area inside where psychics feel a strong radiating current of chi energy flowing upward. Undoubtedly this site holds many secrets yet to be uncovered as we learn more about our ancestors knowledge.

The Four Corners, USA

Sacred ground to the Navajo Indians, the Four Corners got its name from the four states from which it is composed - Utah, Colorado, New Mexico and Arizona. This is a place where you can meet with the Creator in sacred prayer and ceremony, since so much intense prayer energy has been "gathered" here. Once a year there is a huge pow wow which increases the power of the site. There have also been several enormous New Age gatherings here in the past few years (approx. 100,000 people attend).

Mt. Shasta, USA

A mountain of the Gods, there is an inner city within this mountain where ancient Lemurians are said to live as well as members of the White Brotherhood. This location is a powerful transformative emotional vortex. It is also an interdimensional vortex where you can travel into the mountain. You will notice a profound difference in yourself once you leave!

Garden of the Gods, USA

These red rocks pop up on the slopes of the Colorado Rockies in a most unexpected place. When you enter and stroll around, you know you are on sacred ground. Peace and tranquility descend upon you. The ancient Native Americans of this area honored it as sacred, and their essence and energy lives on in the rocks. The eagles soar above these sacred red rocks and bless it with their presence.

There are so many other wonderful and energy transforming sites worldwide, but I can only mention a few here. Please let me know your experiences, and where you find sacred sites so I can share the information with others.

The key to enjoying Mother Earth is in learning to sensitize your body to her energy fields so you can locate special places close to home which will rejuvenate and assist you on your path.

There are many books available on this topic so you can research power points in your area, but watch for an upcoming publication called, *Planetary Influences*, which will be available from my publisher.

Like our bodies, where the veins carry our blood and our unseen energy lines carry our energy, the ley lines of Mother Earth connect many places in an unseen way. It is said that Glastonbury is connected to Mt. Shasta. It is said that the Big Island of Hawaii is connected to Ireland and New Zealand. In this way, ancient people sent energy and communicated with those far away.

One of the most famous ley lines is the St. Michael line which comes up out of the Atlantic onto English soil at Land's End, Cornwall and travels across England, linking up many ancient sites.

A retired New Zealand pilot has gathered massive data about the likelihood that UFO's travel around our planet on ley lines. Sightings have been mapped for years by this man, whose theory is that —in some way—UFOs use our planet's grid as energy highways for their travel.

Herbs, Healing Plants & Homeopathy

This book would not be complete without mentioning that there is a cure for almost every malady available in the forests and fields of Mother Earth.

So much has been written about various herbs for healing that I am not going to go into any great detail here. It is a source of remedies that all of us should be aware of before using lab-created drugs.

The Native Americans and all indigenous people knew where to gather the plants they needed for curing their people. It is pleasing to see more and more interest in this sacred science today.

The flower remedies and the potent liquid

extracts you can now purchase in any health food store are very beneficial not only on a physical level but on an energetic and emotional level as well.

At the same time we are destroying our rain forests, we are also benefiting more than ever before by the plants being discovered in the rain forests. I have even heard that some of the old medicine people in the tribes along the Amazon basin are able to bring plants into our dimension by reaching into the fifth dimension and manifesting them back to us even after we destroyed them on this physical level.

Personally, I am a great believer in using Echinachea and Golden Seal to keep the immune system high. Ginseng is excellent for added vitality and lots of Vitamin C.

I strongly urge you to seek out natural enhancers for your good health.

Crystals & Minerals

The Cherokee Nation considers crystals to be the brain cells of Mother Earth. When we realize that man has now figured out how to make computers work and clocks tick based on crystal energies, we may begin to realize that the ancient Cherokees perhaps knew more about the power of the crystal than we were led to believe.

There is also much information available for reading about the role crystals and other minerals played in the ancient civilizations of Atlantis and

Lemuria. While many do not believe these places ever existed, others like myself know from past life recall that not only did they exist, but that crystals indeed played a large role in day to day life there. If you are interested in reading more information about Atlantis and the crystal connection there, Edgar Cayce covered these topics quite extensively in some of his books, which are available from A.R.E. in Virginia Beach, Virginia.

There are crystal cities on many other planets and star systems. Venus has a crystal city which is at least seventh dimensional energy and therefore unable to be seen by our eyes. There was a crystal planet as well, inhabited by crystal people. Murry Hope's two books, *The Lion People* and *The Paschats and the Crystal People* give a fascinating insight into these beings.

It is my belief, as well as that of many other people who work with and love crystals and minerals, that these precious beings were gifted to our planet. They can be used in healing, beautification and also in communication with other places in this universe and beyond.

A large portion of this book is given over to crystal and mineral knowledge gathered by me during years of experimentation.

The
Element
of
WATER

Healing Waters, Sacred Springs & Wells

The beneficial aspects of healing waters have been known throughout history, and many people have gone to "take the waters" over the centuries in Europe either for healing or rejuvenation.

In Great Britain it has been speculated that many of the ancient wells were positioned either on a ley line, or at the end of a ley line. This could account for the powerful healing properties found in the waters of some of the ancient wells, as well as the minerals found in the water itself.

Below are just a few of the many global locations, some of which are better known than others, where you will find sacred waters for your body, mind, spirit and emotions. If you know of sacred or healing waters in your area, please send me the information so I can pass it on to others.

Chalice Well, England

The waters of Chalice Well, near Glastonbury, England, are located in one of England's most sacred areas, steeped in mystery and mystical events, and associated with the times of Camelot, Merlin, Lancelot, Guinevere, King Arthur and the Knights of the Round Table.

There is so much iron in the water, it creates a reddish color, and therefore many call it the Blood Well. This also led to the legend that the Holy Grail is located in the depths of the well and that Christ's blood is what causes the waters to be reddish. There are two streams of water–one is said to be clear and the other red. This water is only available for healing in the form of drinking water from the Chalice Well Gardens.

Its properties are excellent for spiritual cleansing and emotional expansion. There are also case histories available of physical healings.

The origin of these waters is still a mystery, but we know they come from a place of inner purity, innocence and emotional well being from deep within Mother Earth.

One of the most pleasing and sacred encounters I can recommend is a meditation in Chalice Well Gardens, which would empower you with strength and peace. Choose your spot, settle down and connect with the tranquility of the area. While there, I connected with the transformative, loving and gentle energy of Venus, which can be strongly felt there.

The Healing Hole, North Bimini, Bahamas

In contrast, the reward of bathing in the waters of the Healing Hole on Bimini comes as a result of a pilgrimage, of sorts, which you must be willing to undertake. A small boat with a local navigator will ferry you at top speed through the mangroves in order to access the remote Healing Hole. You will disembark on a shallow sandbar, in what seems to be the middle of nowhere, and must then walk through the water in order to reach your destination.

These waters contain many minerals, and appear to have a high content of lithium, which balances the body and mind and brings peace of mind. Lithium is one of the drugs used to treat schizophrenia and other mental illnesses, so this natural spring, which is available to all, is very theraputic.

This sacred spot was originally "located" by Edgar Cayce during a reading for one of his clients who subsequently flew to Bimini and discovered its location.

There are small metaphysical tours which go to Bimini to experience the many mysteries this small island has to offer. The world famous Row of Stones, considered by many to be part of old Atlantis rising, was first discovered psychically by Edgar Cayce in a reading.

Energy-sensitive people will be amazed by the whole energy field of this island, which, in spite of it being part of the Bahamas, feels neither Bahamian nor American (nearest neighbor), but "otherworldly." To feel it is to believe it.

There is an excellent video, *Mysteries of Bimini, When Spirits Come Calling*, which I can recommend if you are interested in a trip to Bimini; it will show you the mystical sites, including a trip to the healing hole, so you know what you can expect before going, (see details at the back of this book). I've been on an excellent tour, run by Gwen at Dolphin Discovery World Tours. Her tours go to many metaphysical destinations worldwide and her Bimini trip is extraordinary.

Australian "Waterholes"

The healing waters of Australia are not internationally well known, but as usual the natives of any country know where to find them.

The Aborigines consider many waterholes as sacred throughout their land. Some of the ones that are not secretly guarded are possibly accessible to all, however, in respect to the Aborigines and their beliefs, you should ask before entering the waters.

According to a recent TV program on the Discovery Channel, there is an area in Australia where the cattle are living to be twice their age, and are still reproducing at 18 and 20 years old, which is not considered a normal age for reproduction. Scientists are intrigued and have tested everything the cattle are exposed to in order to discover the source of their vitality. They have decided the secret is in the spring water the cattle are drinking, which is so loaded with minerals that the ranchers don't drink it!

Kulunbar (Katherine Gorge), Australia

This area is located in Jawoyn country in the Northern Territory. Like many of the sacred water-holes, it is connected with the rainbow snake, who is said to have carved the gorge with his body. The river winds to the sacred hot springs of Mataranka in the south and the Douglas hot springs in the north.

There are other sacred water locations around the world; the natives are the best people to ask since they have always strongly relied on natural healing sources.

Abalone

Abalone is a shell instead of a mineral, so I am including it in this section. It is one of the most beautiful gifts Mother Nature has given us from the water element, as well as pearls.

When it comes to healing, it is the emotional body which is transformed by working with this luminous, colorful shell. It is like the opal of the water world.

To enhance your psychic abilities, it is recommended that you get an abalone sphere, obelisk or pyramid to work with. Tune into the water kingdom through meditation.

More connected with the Pacific Ocean and Ancient Lemuria than with Atlantis, it carries the memories of gentle offerings and whale and dolphin communications. These were the times when humans and their water world relatives celebrated together. Tuning in to abalone can also increase your ability to communicate with these water mammals.

Several Native American tribes, especially those living near the coastal regions, used the abalone shell as the sacred vessel in which sage and other herbs were burned in special offerings. This is the union of fire and water, which creates sacred smoke. When you are performing a ceremony like this, with love in your heart, you are providing the ether of love which is the catalyst for transformation.

It is a shame that man has polluted the oceans and waterways of our world with dangerous chemicals. The ocean creatures are struggling to survive. The cycle of the food chain is being disrupted because we are now eating contaminated seafood. Making a prayer offering to bless the creatures and mammals and purify the oceans will promote healing on the unseen planes.

Elixirs

The basic description of an elixir is a "potion" you drink made from steeping specific minerals in purified water. This can be very beneficial and theraputic for your body and mind, but before preparing any elixir, you must do your research and make sure you are not working with stones which are either toxic or poisonous! Most mineral books would supply the information you need, or consult your local rock expert. If in doubt, don't do it. It may be hazardous to your health.

My favorite elixir is made with moldavite, which you can read about in the moldavite section on page 75. I often make a gallon and drink it throughout the month. This is an excellent way to learn more about your vibrational sensitivity and to heighten your extrasensory perception.

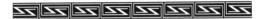

The
Element
of
FIRE

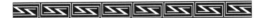

Solar & Volcanic Energies

Both of these energies are fire; one is internal and the other is external. Solar energy comes from the heavens while volcanic energy comes from the core of Mother Earth herself.

The sun has been worshipped as the supreme God by many ancient peoples around the world since the beginning of time. The power of heat and light given off by this ball of fire are responsible for life on this planet, and there is no question that without the sun we would not have life on Earth.

Various indigenous tribes like the Mayans, Incas and Egyptians all worshipped the Sun God. Light made crop growth possible, and warmed the lands to a temperature at which human life could survive. The production of chlorophyll which makes plants green could not take place without the Sun. Oxygen, therefore, would not be available without the sun's rays.

Many decades of abuse by humans in the form of chemical dumping, toxic waste, nuclear incidents and general carelessness has caused a great imbalance on Mother Earth. One of the many results is dangerous holes in the ozone layer which now allow unfiltered sunlight to enter in a global warming effect. As a result, Australia and Chile to name just two countries, are suffering high rates of blindness and skin cancer and in Australia school children must wear sunglasses and hats to school.

Volcanic energy, while usually viewed as destructive, actually creates the most fertile land on which a rich multitude of flora and crops can be grown after many years of cooling.

Kundalini

Mother Earth's volcanic eruptions are similar to human kundalini energy, whereby we consciously invoke our energies to rise from deep within.

Pele is the goddess of volcanoes and is respected and feared by Hawaiians who know her power.

When we learn not to be afraid of our own internal power surges and emotional eruptions, we will also learn not to fear the unknown in our lives. Then we can transmute fear to respect. A meditation focusing on volcanic energy can help us face and overcome these fearful emotions.

When you are in your emotional power, you can be in the eye of a hurricane or the path of a tornado and remain safe and untouched. The key is in Knowing.

Candles

Burning candles is another ceremonial tool which has been used for centuries around the world. Not only does the candle bring light into the darkness, but it also symbolizes the heat of the Sun and the fire of transmutation. It helps you focus on visualization techniques.

When you work with candles as described in this book, remember to place each candle—no matter what color the candle is—in a white dish with water in it. The water serves to magnify the power of the candle, and therefore your intention. Water is also a conductor, and will carry your intention where it needs to go. White represents purity and is all encompassing.

Burning a candle intensifies your aims. As you read this book, you will find many suggestions about how to use candles in connection with various healing and meditative practices.

As with many tools, the more meaning you put into it, the more you will receive from it. Choosing the most appropriately colored candle and focusing your intent will give you stronger results.

The
Element of
ETHER

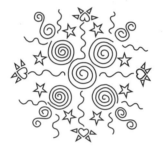

Sacred
Synthesis

The Element of Ether

The main components of the element Ether are vibrations and frequencies of love and light. Love is the cohesive glue that holds our universe and our reality together. Love is the healing power behind everything.

We are most familiar with frequencies and vibrations in the forms of color, light and sound. Each color carries a vibrational tone, and each sound carries a physical vibration. In ancient societies such as Atlantis, the healing temples were mostly color and sound oriented.

Crystals, as conductors and transmitters, can be charged and programmed to carry any frequency and vibration, which makes them of invaluable assistance to fifth dimensional healers.

Crystal bowls are a great way to combine crystal energy with sound. There are seven bowls for the seven main chakras, or energy wheels of the body, and each has its own vibration and sound. These are excellent for aligning your chakras and getting you in tune with sound healing.

You will always find harmony and healing by becoming conscious of the colors and sounds you surround yourself with. Windchimes, bells and harmonious music will work to heal you without you even knowing it! Experiments have shown that harp music heals many ailments with its celestial sounds.

Feng Shui, the ancient Chinese art of placement, is just one of many teachings which respects the importance of appropriate use of color for creating a harmonious environment.

If you are nervous and hyper, for instance, don't wear red or have a lot of red in your rooms. You need blue, green or muted pastels to calm you down. If you are lethargic, you need reds, oranges and bold colors to activate you.

A little studying of Feng Shui and Sacred Geometry will enhance your understanding of how everything is connected within the secret workings of our universe.

Synthesis

The whole is greater than the sum of its parts. The fifth element, Ether, provides the alchemical bonding which transmutes the other four elements of Air, Earth, Fire and Water. The fifth component creates a new "One" and activates it into a more potent healing form than any of the single elements. This is the icing on the cake, or the holographic perfection that is there for us to tap into if we consciously work toward this goal.

You can walk up to a sacred spring and see it as only water; you can pick up a crystal lying at your feet and see it only as a stone; you can hear music and tune it out. Yet, when you combine the essence of these elements as a form of consciousness and explore how you can utilize the mysteries within them, then you see everything with new eyes and create a new reality of wellness for yourself. This is the Magic of Love. This will take you into fifth dimensional living and healing.

Just like we have five physical senses, we have the five elements described above. There is a healing aspect to each of our senses. The sixth sense is equal to the total of the five elements because once they are combined they become the ultimate element. *Again I say, the whole is greater than the sum of its parts.*

The more we focus on Love, the brighter our light bodies will grow. We will become luminous and will emanate love on all levels. Then we are fifth dimensional healers.

Healthy mind.
Healthy body.
Healthy emotions.
Healthy spirit.

Love is I AM.

Love

Love is the ether of life and controls all our emotions. It is the healer of everything. Like food and water, without love we cannot survive, and with love we can soar to the greatest heights. It is the key and the gateway to everything. It will align all your chakras in harmony. When you do *anything* with love in your heart, it changes the outcome; it is the ultimate catalyst.

When working with crystals and minerals, opening your heart chakra and connecting with your higher self makes the difference between a successful experience and a disappointing one. Like the petals of the rose, love is soft and gentle.

Many people say they cannot feel the vibration of a crystal when they hold it, and I always tell them to open their hearts so the love vibration can be the link. Those who let go of their fears and vulnerabilities long enough to attempt this are amazed at the power of love. In this way, we learn to trust again and this, in itself, is a healing.

If you can bring yourself to send love to those who have hurt you the deepest, you will be rewarded with love in return. Often, by sending love to those who wish you no good, you can turn the energy of the situation around to a positive outcome.

Always remember that you cannot love another being successfully until you have first learned to love yourself. Give your inner child a lot of love so she or he can be healed.

Love is multidimensional, ranging from the divine to the passionate. It is the purest and most unconditional form of love which we need to tap into for alchemical transformation. The lesser forms of love, such as the heat of passion, are temporary and don't have the strength and endurance of divine love.

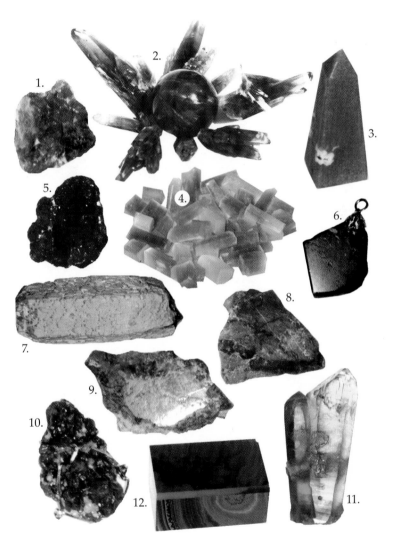

1) Alexandrite 2) Amethyst 3) Angelite 4) Ulexite 5) Azurite
6) Bloodstone 7) Candle Quartz 8) Sugilite 9) Chrysocolla
10) Cinnabar 11) Citrine 12) Malachite

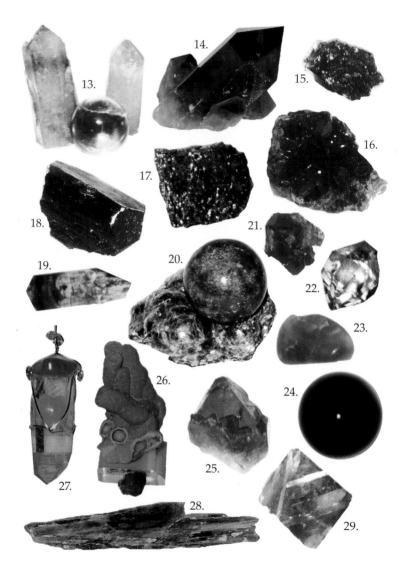

13) Quartz 14) Smokey Quartz 15) Moldavite 16) Dioptase 17) Galena
18) Black Tourmaline 19) Watermelon Tourmaline 20) Lepidolite
21) Green Garnet 22) Herkimer Diamond 23) Aventurine 24) Obsidian Ball
25) Strawberry Quartz 26) Rhodochrosite 27) Love Power Pack
28) Blue Kyanite 29) Purple Flourite

Part II

The Crystal People

Cleansing Your Crystal

Much has been written about this subject, so I'll say very little. There is only one true way to cleanse a crystal, and that is through vibration. Brass chimes, which are yin & yang, the tone of a crystal quartz tuning bowl, or striking a tuning fork are the best ways to remove negativity from your crystal or mineral.

Smudging and salt water, or holding it under running water and burying it, all cleanse to a lesser degree, only affecting the surface and leaving the internal body of the crystal contaminated. Marcel Vogel, one of the greatest pioneers of scientific experiments involving crystal energy, found this to be true in his lab.

The crystals and minerals that you are now a keeper of, took millions and millions of years to find you. They are Earth's treasures, having been hidden in her heart since the beginning of time. What an honor and privilege it is to have one as your special friend and companion.

You may come upon a crystal that was with you before in a past life, and experience an awareness of previously having been together. Now you are reunited; give your crystal love and you will receive love in return. Your new friend will help you in so many ways. The feeling is wonderful and special.

You are the Keeper of the Crystal during this

lifetime, so honor it. It is full of information and power which it might share with you if you learn to love it.

Crystal Enlightenment Through Crystal & Mineral Healing

Below you will find what I believe are magical combinations of various crystals and minerals which I have tested while working with many people worldwide over the years. The results have spoken for themselves and therefore I wish to share this information with you.

When working with the various crystals and minerals, also keep in mind which colors you are working with. Just as the rainbow contains the energies of all the colors, the specific colors of the minerals hold healing powers as well.

Alexandrite

Recently I had the good fortune to come across some very rare Russian alexandrite crystals in the matrix from the Ural Mountains. Even though they are very costly and hard to come by, I want to share this information with you in case you find some available. Alexandrite has a color change from green to deep red and the colors of the crystal are very intense.

While meditating with them in my hands, I could feel such a strong vibration from them. The intensity of the crystals made it feel like my hands were magnets and that I couldn't open them even if I tried. I didn't want to open them and didn't want the experience to end. The calmness and serenity this experience gave me was very powerful. I felt the magnetic pull of the stones could lead me through a portal into the future.

Alexandrite was much more readily available several decades ago, and I've heard of more than one person finding some of these costly stones in antique rings at flea markets and pawn shops at great bargain prices. The sellers didn't seem to know the value of what they had.

Amethyst Phantom

An amethyst phantom removes anger, depression, addictions and other negative states of emotion. On a physical level, it helps remove heart problems in some circumstances.

When there are baby points inside of an amethyst phantom, it takes on the very powerful properties of being a Manifestation tool. A manifestation crystal of any kind brings the special gift of knowing how to assist you in manifesting what you want to bring into your life.

When working with amethysts in general for healing or spiritual purposes, lighting a purple candle before you begin can enhance your results. The candle and the mineral both vibrate to the frequency of the color purple, and as we know, color is a visual translation of vibration.

Case History

A man in his late fifties with heart valve complications came to have healing treatments. He was laid out with crystals, and a phantom amethyst was waved over his heart area twenty-one times. This removed the pain he was feeling, and upon his next visit to the doctor, he was looking and feeling well again. The doctor commented on his better state of health.

Angelite

Named for the angels, it is a soft blue quartz, wonderful to hold and feel, and emits a soft vibration. Try it on your third eye when you meditate. It is so peaceful and calming, it will leave you with the feeling that you are floating on air, just like an angel.

For an even deeper experience, light a blue candle and surround yourself with purple light. Add a piece of apophyllite over each eyelid at the same time, and enjoy the angelic trip.

This would be an excellent time to communicate with your guardian angel or birth right angel, and to draw the angelic energies into your own sphere for daily strength and guidance. If you have not met your angel yet, ask him or her to show themselves to you during an angelite meditation.

Apophyllite & Ulexite

Apophyllite is a clear crystal that is pyramidal in shape. It is excellent for focussing your third eye during meditation, and for healing the eyes of redness, tiredness, strain, and computer-related exposure.

Apophyllite is an "otherworldly" stone, and some of the most beautiful and mystical pieces originate in India. The sea green variety is extremely magical and works very well in oceanic meditations and connecting with the undersea world and lost civilizations.

Hold ulexite in your hand, as it works powerfully to assist apophyllite as a booster, "kicking it in" for more intense results. Based on many years of experience, ulexite has proven itself to be an enhancer for use with other minerals and crystals.

Ulexite will also help you get more in tune with any stones that you hold. When testing for sensitivity of various stones within your own personal energy field, use a small piece of ulexite in your receiving hand, and the other stone or mineral in your other hand. Allow three to five minutes. You will be amazed at the heightened vibrations you will be able to feel from both hands. Everybody is different, and while some are extremely sensitive to stone vibrations, others need assistance and long term exposure to minerals in order to build their sensitivity.

Azurite

This beautiful cosmic blue crystal is good for high energy, meditation, and the American Natives used it for telepathic communication.

Along with blue kyanite, it is very good for the throat chakra and for sore throats and laryngitis.

When working with this combination, light a dark blue candle.

"As-you-write" or azurite, promotes creative writing and thinking. This operates through telepathic communication, and the deep blue color of azurite assists in connecting with universal consciousness.

I gave a piece of azurite to my friend Gwen as a gift while she was writing her new book. She told me it greatly enhanced her creativity while writing the manuscript and literally influenced the flow, whereby the name "as-you-write" developed.

Bloodstone & Sugilite

This is a wonderful combination for thinning the blood, rejuvenating the blood for people who suffer from heart problems, and physical and internal problems.

Bloodstone is great for women during menustration if they are afflicted with cramps, severe bleeding, clots, or other known related menstral problems.

Bloodstone also assists those suffering from hemorrhoids, and the sugilite helps to remove pain and swelling. Keep it close to your body, holding it in your hands, or wearing it.

This combination is excellent for the physical body, and everybody can benefit from it as a preventative external "blood tonic" not taken internally.

Candle Quartz

Also known as the Magician's Stone, candle quartz is a magical stone with good vibrations. It can be used in conjunction with several other stones for excellent effects, mostly for meditation.

For this meditation experience, you will need 12 pieces of moldavite, a candle quartz, a clear quartz, and four white candles. Surround yourself with the pink light of love and feel love emanating from your heart chakra.

Place the four candles to the north, south, east and west, and align yourself with head facing east.

You are pulling in universal energies with the moldavite. Omitting thumb/forefinger and Big toe/index toe, place a piece of moldavite between all your other fingers and toes. Then hold a candle quartz in your receiving (left) hand and a clear quartz in your sending (right) hand. Enjoy the experience; it is truly unique.

If there are interdimensional or intergalactic beings you wish to connect with, the combination of candle quartz and moldavite can help you call these beings into your sphere.

Chrysocolla

All sugar-related problems benefit from chrysocolla. This can range from sugar and chocolate cravings to diabetes. You must hold the stone or have it on your body at all times (a wire wrapped pendant or earring would be good). Experience has shown that the blood sugar count returns to normal when a piece of chrysocolla is worn constantly. However, as with all physical illnesses mentioned throughout this book, you must continue to consult with your doctor.

Case History

Bob, a very close family friend, is a six and a half foot tall biker and tattoo artist. He came to me with diabetes, and his sugar count was excessively high. I wrapped a piece of chrysocolla for him to wear as an earring, and within a few days, his sugar count returned to normal. From time to time crises that arise in his life make his count go out of whack again, but he has had a lot of success managing it with his chrysocolla earring.

All sugar related problems reflect a craving for love, or a lack of sweetness in your life. Take time to dwell on the issue of love and see if you can locate the problem. This can help repattern your inner love chords and go a long way toward healing sugar-related problems, too.

Cinnabar, Malachite & Citrine

Used in combination, this is a powerful tool to bring financial abundance and prosperity to yourself. Cinnabar is deep red, with glittering flakes of crystal, and is very "rich" looking; citrine is like liquid gold, and malachite is green which is the color of money in our society. Therefore, on a color vibration level as well, this combination is very potent for prosperity.

You are also working here again with the power of three and the fact that the whole is greater than the sum of its parts.

As with using all stones to assist in achieving our desires, the more you focus on how these stones can assist in your particular case, the more potent will be the outcome.

Citrine & Amber

This combination is very good for improving the function of your urinary system, and can assist in cleansing your kidneys for optimum use.

Light a yellow or gold candle, in your bedroom, and sleep with citrine and amber in your hands.

Some say that drinking amber tea, an elixir, assists women with fertility problems to overcome them and become pregnant. I cannot say I have known of such a case personally, but if this is your issue, you may wish to try a cup of amber tea.

Amber is a great conductor of energy between you and the tree spirits. It will assist you in tuning in to them, and you can ask for elemental energy to give you a physical boost if you are running on low steam.

Crystal Quartz Clusters & Black Tourmaline

Clear or milky, crystal quartz clusters are excellent for placing under a bed to get rid of unwanted entities and energies. Place one cluster in the attic (if you have one) and one cluster under your bed. They can be small clusters, since size is not equal to potency.

At the same time, put black tourmalines in all four corners of the room to get rid of unwanted negativity. Black tourmaline is the strongest stone for blocking and ridding your environment of negative energy. It is the equalizer, or bouncer, of the stone world.

Smudge your home or apartment with sage. Try to get the purest and highest quality sage which is in silver, long leaf form. Don't forget to cleanse yourself at the same time.

Following such a ceremony your sacred space will be free of negativity and stale energy, refreshed and ready for you to fill with positive and creative ideas once again.

Dioptase & Moldavite

Dioptase is the deepest emerald green and has such a smooth, calming feeling to it. Try holding a piece of dioptase in your left, receiving hand, with a piece of moldavite in your right (sending) hand. It is like time traveling to a forest in outer space.

Light a green candle in advance, and surround yourself with universal energy and call upon Venus for guidance. It's like being somewhere in time, but not knowing where. This is an excellent way to travel interdimensionally.

Dioptase holds many secrets of the heart and of the rainforests within the depths of its green crystals. Your eyes can experience healing energy entering your body, by staring at a piece of deeply green colored dioptase. Consciously "pull" the green deep into your eyes and, in meditation, let the green light energy travel to your heart chakra. Feel the healing energy emit love waves to empower your heart to greater compassion.

Galena

For anybody working with radiology, as well as computer operators and anybody exposed to harmful electro-magnetic frequencies coming from a machine in their vicinity, I highly recommend galena. For those working in a job where they are operating machinery which gives off these frequencies or radioactive frequencies, even if you have protective environments, you should carry a piece of galena in your pocket to counteract this energy. Galena pulls radiation to it and away from you. It will also gradually remove it from you if you have been exposed to it in the past.

Likewise if you are working all day on a computer, or watch a lot of TV, you are exposed to harmful rays. By placing a piece of galena on top of your monitor or TV and preferably another piece below it, this will scatter the waves which otherwise emanate in your direction.

I have two pieces on my own computer and after two years they are eroding in certain places where the negative energies have been absorbed into the galena.

I have wondered if it would comfort chemo and radiology patients and possibly ease their side effects if they carried a piece of galena with them. It certainly wouldn't hurt them, so if anybody has any feedback on this, please let me know (this is not medical advice).

Luckily galena is easy to find and very inexpensive.

Case History

After working with a woman who came to the crystal shop looking for some stones, she gave me a hug before leaving. I immediately got dizzy and had to sit down; I felt very strange. I asked her where she worked. She told me she was a nurse in radiology. I explained to her the effect she had on me, and that she was very toxic. I gave her a piece of galena to carry on her. She came back to the store two weeks later and told me she felt better than she had in ages. She sent ten more nurses to me to get galena!

Green Garnet & Sugilite

Green garnet: is very good for back pain and lower back problems. It has a very strong vibration, and works excellently with a piece of sugilite, which eases pain. Combined, they are a double dose working in harmony together.

It has been said that green garnet is excellent for legal matters and court battles. As an experiment, a friend of mine who had multiple court cases within a few month period, took a green garnet to court on every occasion, and won at every court appearance! Three of these appearances were on "Friday the 13ths". Based on this, I feel the stone has significant powers in the line of upholding justice. However, don't expect the stone to help you win in court if you have not been truthful, since it is an enforcer of justice.

Herkimer Diamonds
& Apophyllite

For deep meditation, surround yourself in a circle of crystals. Place a piece of apophyllite on your third eye, and put a herkimer in each hand. Light a white candle and surround yourself with white light. Call upon your spiritual guides for guidance and keep love in your heart.

For those who have difficulty getting into a meditative state, this will make it easier to let go and let God/Goddess come in and the everyday clutter of your thoughts to go away.

Kunzite

Lavender kunzite is a wonderful stone for love, telepathic communication and for manifesting your dreams and desires.

When working with kunzite, light a pink candle and focus your energies on what you love and desire. If you are working with a photograph of a person or thing, placing a piece of kunzite on the photo will manifest your intentions. If you don't have a photo, you can write a description on a piece of white plain paper and then place the kunzite on top. You will be amazed at the results. Remember, the more focused you are, the quicker your results will be. However, everything happens in its own time, so be patient and know that what is yours will come to you. Always be careful what you ask for, you just might get it!

Case History

Many people have come to me over the years suffering from grief, whether it is over the loss of their mate, a pet or a sudden sense of lonliness. Every time this happens, I find the best remedy is to recommend love stones to them. There are many to choose from, and of course all crystals are full of love. However, there are a few "specialists" such as rose quartz, lavender kunzite, strawberry quartz and amethyst. If you let them, they will love you. If you are grieving or lonely you can fill the gap within yourself with the love vibrations of these crystals. Turn up your self love and use the special affirmation, "I AM LOVE."

Lepidolite & Tourmaline

This combination promotes a focused mind, especially when you are studying and need to memorize information.

Lepidolite has a soft, lavender color to it and you can meditate with it to train your mind not to wander and give way to scattered thoughts. Simply hold it in one of your hands while studying with the intent to retain the information.

Tourmaline comes in a variety of colors, but in this case it is the green tourmaline that works most effectively.

Light a lavender colored candle when working with it, and use some lavender oils to enhance the air you breathe during your study period. Also make sure you have enough fresh air to breathe and light to see by.

This combination not only helps you focus on what you are learning, it also strengthens your ability to retain information and draw on it when necessary. It is excellent for students of all ages.

Malachite & Aventurine

If you wish to bring prosperity into your life, get a piece each of malachite and aventurine and keep them close to you. Light a green candle under the full moon with the intention of attracting more prosperity to yourself. Surround yourself with white light and have love in your heart.

Don't forget that the heart chakra color is green, and that by expanding your love consciousness you will automatically increase your abundance.

If you can get a manifestation crystal, which is a crystal with a "baby" crystal growing inside, this is a very powerful tool for increasing abundance, or anything else you decide to manifest in your life.

There are many forms of prosperity and abundance, not all of which are financial. Perhaps your abundance is in the form of a rewarding job or a loving relationship, or expansion of your psychic abilities. Learn to value non-material forms of abundance, in addition to the rewards of the physical world, for a happy life.

Moldavite

I feel that moldavite is a very powerful protector, healer and is a sacred stone from outer space that has come to us by the guidance of The Creator.

Moldavite can be used as an elixir as long as it is placed under the full moon in a natural crystal glass which contains no lead. Mountain spring water should be used.

From personal experience, it has helped women with fertility problems, and drinking moldavite-charged water has helped many women with anorexia and bulimia to overcome their lack of self love, in combination with Reiki healings. It is an excellent protector against misfortune, and will keep you out of harm's way. The definition of harm's way can be as deadly as a car crash or as seemingly minor as a speeding ticket. It will forewarn you in a very strange way to protect you. The key is in listening to it; a warning is only useful if you listen to it and act on it.

Moldavite is a spiritual enhancer in a power pack (see section on Power Packs). It is very good for third eye meditation and is a powerful healing tool when placed between the fingers while doing hands on healing. Be very careful how you do this; always ask for Creator's guidance and universal wisdom. Personally, I call on Venus and tap into universal love, which is an endless source of energy, when I do healing sessions.

I highly recommend that Reiki Masters and other hands-on healers use six pieces of moldavite between their fingers (three for each hand, all but thumb/forefinger positions) when doing healing work. The moldavite enhances the ability to transform the person's energy field to a more positive and healthier vibration.

Choose one of the following three to surround the individual you are working with: clear quartz, red phantom crystals, or green fluorite crystals. Do not mix the above, since each has its own powerful focus. Cleanse your crystals before or after each treatment.

Light a red candle to enhance the energetic healing, and call upon the universal energies of Venus and ask for God's guidance.

Moldavite & Ulexite

To stimulate Moldavite to a higher level of vibration, use a piece of ulexite with it. It acts as a catalyst and intensifies the effect you can expect from moldavite.

Moldavite between the fingers is very good for removing arthritis pains. Sleep with it at night between the fingers; if you have difficulty, use cotton gloves to keep the stones in place, or some medical tape. You will notice the difference.

Case History

An eighty year old woman with arthritic fingers was in such a state that her hands had closed up into fists. She could no longer open them freely. A piece of moldavite was placed into the closed palm of each hand, and by morning her hands were open and operating normally once more, after four years of suffering. Three years later the condition had not reappeared and she continues to enjoy healthy and agile hands.

Obsidian

Obsidian and clear quartz work well for those who wish to contact beings on the other side. Whether you wish to call in spirits in general or use a tool such as table tipping, the pendulum or channeling, begin by placing a piece of obsidian under your left foot and a quartz crystal under your right foot. This is because your left foot is the receiver, and obsidian will ground you; your right foot is the sender, and quartz crystal is a communication tool. Ground yourself and surround yourself with white light as you call in the universal energies and your angels, guides and teachers.

To eliminate a personal problem, no matter what it may be, you should use a black obsidian sphere with a silver sheen on the top and bottom. Write your problem very clearly on a piece of paper and put it under the sphere. Leave it alone and keep it in a place where it won't be disturbed. For optimal results, do this at the time of the full moon, at midnight. Light a black candle in a white dish with water and let it burn out. Walk away and forget about the problem, turning it over to the obsidian to handle. Your problem will usually resolve itself.

Remember the univeral laws of cause and effect when deciding to use this tool. Never use it in a manner that will cause harm to another, or surely the boomerang will swing around and hit you. What you send out always comes back to you as well.

Purple Fluorite

We all have good days and bad days, but when you have a real bad day and get to the point of blowing up, or coming unglued, grab a piece of purple fluorite and hold it with both hands. Relax with it, close your eyes, and feel the anger and tension leave your body through the help of the fluorite. You'll be amazed how it will work with you to bring you back to a state of gentle calmness.

Sleeping Disorders: When you cannot fall asleep, light a pink candle and hold a piece of purple fluorite. Surround yourself with pink light. Be still. In your mind tell yourself to be still twenty-one times. You will fall asleep. Remember, the magic phrase is, "be still."

You can also put a piece of ulexite or clear quartz in one of your hands while still holding the fluorite, and surround yourself with purple or lavender light and enjoy the calmness.

This combination is excellent for stress reduction.

Rhodochrosite

This love stone comes in varying shades of red, from almost orange to a deeper rose-red color. It often has white or cream colored veins which can be circular or spiral-shaped, and is a very beautiful crystal. It is often used for jewelery.

I create love power packs with rhodochrosite when it is the heart chakra that needs to be open and receptive. This stone represents unconditional love, and is usually wrapped with a pure quartz crystal point to accelerate the opening of the heart chakra.

As you will read in this book, rose quartz, strawberry quartz and kunzite are other love stones. All of these crystals and stones are in the pink to red spectrum, which relate to different sorts of love, from the innocent and pure to the passionate.

In my experience, there are several love categories: spiritual love, innocent and pure love, unconditional love and passionate love. Each of these love crystals is most aligned with one of these categories:

Kunzite is passionate, interpersonal love.
Rose Quartz is innocent and pure love.
Rhodocrosite is the heart of love.
Strawberry Quartz is unconditional, cosmic
  love.

Strawberry Quartz Rutilated with Lepidolite

This is a beautiful love stone to work with. It is from Russia and is hard to find. I currently have a source for this costly and rare stone, although it is hard to know how long it will be available on the market.

Having worked with it personally and with many other people, I know it has a very unique love vibration to it. It is for unconditional, cosmic love more than interpersonal love.

Sugilite, Moldavite & Ulexite

This is an excellent combination for a person recovering from surgery. You can either place these three stones on the recovering area of the body, or simply hold them in your hands. They have a powerful effect by diminishing pain in an accelerated manner.

When working with these minerals, lighting a green and a white candle is complimentary and will enhance the results you may expect.

Sugilite, Purple Fluorite & Blue Kyanite

When working with any amount of stones, make sure they are all touching your body at the same time. If they are small you can hold them in your hands, otherwise good places for them are on your chakra areas.

Sugilite can be used as an excellent pain remover and healer placed over the affected area. It will remove discomfort in a matter of five to twenty minutes depending on the pain intensity. It is excellent for menstrual cramps. In the case of fevers, it literally drains the fever from your body. Sugilite has a high content of manganese in it, and this is the mineral that pulls pain right out of your body.

At the same time you can use it combined with purple fluorite and blue kyanite. All three minerals combined together will work as a powerful healing device, especially for flu-like symptoms such as fever and stress. Fluorite and kyanite are excellent together to take away hypertension and anxiety attacks. This combination is a mood-enhancing stimulant. Hold one stone in each hand.

The fluorite must be deep purple in color, without any other colors (fluorite comes in many colors).

Kyanite should be the blue variety (it comes in blue, green and black). It is very good to be used for your throat chakra and will remove a sore throat. It is excellent to meditate and sleep with, just like sugilite.

This combination is excellent when dealing with flu and fever. This ties in with the indigo spectrum of color, and therefore if you can, light an indigo candle; it will be beneficial to light it before working with these stones.

These minerals are a gift from Mother Earth to us that we may use as healing tools. Always remember that love is the language you need to use when communicating with the stone people in the crystal and mineral kingdoms. They are wise and know how they can best assist you during your times of need. Speak to them with love. They come to us from Mother Earth and The Creator.

Power Packs

Created with crystals and minerals from Mother Earth, these are special combinations I put together for people depending on what they need to bring into their lives. While I intuitively make power packs on special request, below is a listing of various themes I create for individuals.

Some of my better known power packs are:

> *Vortex of Protection*
> *Love Power Pack*
> *Prosperity Power Pack*
> *Enlightenment Power Pack*
> *Cosmic Power Pack*
> *High Energy Power Pack*
> *Grounding Power Pack*
> *Psychic Power Pack*
> *Manifestation Power Pack*

These power packs are created to assist you. For instance, if you ask for a love power pack, you feel the need to bring more love into your life. Will the power pack be able to manifest this love? Not on its own; the crystals and minerals are there to assist us in obtaining what we are working toward. The right combination of love stones will greatly enhance your abilities to draw love into your life if you are also consciously working within yourself to achieve this result.

I create each and every one of these with love from my heart, and use the healing energies of my hands and my eyes. I surround every crystal with love and light as I build each power pack into a tool for growth and wellbeing. I activate and awaken the crystals on an energetic level so they are ready to work with you. I wrap them either in gold-filled wire or sterling silver, or sometimes both combined, as requested by the person. Each and every creation is a labor of love, and all pieces, upon completion, are cleansed thoroughly.

These power packs are not mass produced or farmed out to third parties, since I need a hands-on approach to alchemically activate the stones.

Crystal Meditation Wheel

To accomplish a strong and clear meditation, create a crystal meditation wheel by surrounding yourself with eight crystal points facing outwards. When the crystals face outwards they release energy from you; when they face inwards, they pull energy in toward you. These eight crystals represent the eight directional points, and the circle represents infinity and the circle of life. Once inside, you can travel anywhere in meditation.

If possible, hold a double terminated quartz point vertically in each hand, so one end points down into Mother Earth and the other up into the universe. This forms a bond between universal energy and Mother Earth energy.

Light four white candles, and place them in the north, south, east and west locations of your crystal meditation wheel. Align your body so your head is facing east when you lie down inside your wheel.

Call upon your spiritual guides to come in to work with you, and to guide your meditation. Allow the crystal people you have surrounded yourself with to still your mind and enhance your meditation.

When your meditation is complete, surround yourself with the white light of truth and protection and pink light of love. Give yourself time to return peacefully to your environment.

Thank the crystals and cleanse them with sound

vibration afterward, and acknowledge the light of the candles which guided your meditation as you blow them out. You can now break the circle.

Copper Pyramids

Here is something I consider an enhancer to crystal work. A copper pyramid frame, made to exact measurements, can be a wonderful tool for deep meditation, raising your frequency and vibration and cleansing you of unwanted energies. In fact, when you sit inside the pyramid, everything you are thinking and feeling will be magnified, so be sure to clear your mind and think only positive thoughts.

A smaller copper pyramid is excellent in the kitchen to purify and lengthen the lifetime of fruits, vegetables, etc. This is an excellent way to purify water and charge it before drinking. It can also intensify the power of elixirs if placed overnight in a pyramid under the light of the full moon. Broken bones have been known to heal quicker if they've been in a pyramid ten to fifteen minutes daily.

About the Author

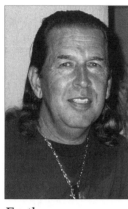

I have been blessed to be able to help many people over the years with physical and emotional problems. They have always found their way to me with God's guidance. I do not charge financially for being able to assist other people, since I consider healing powers to be a gift from the Creator and Mother Earth.

I call upon my Native American guides and ancestors, as well as my power animals and the universal energies when I set about working with crystals. I am an American Native, and very proud of my heritage.

Author Availability

I am available by appointment for the following:

Workshops and seminars. I am also available to travel for these, and request only that all travel-related expenses are covered by the participants.

Personal sessions. I do private energy work on individuals, and you can contact me for more information.

Creating personal power packs. I have been gifted by my guides to be able to reconstruct the DNA of crystals while working with them consciously. I intuitively create the power pack of various minerals and crystals, charged by my own healing powers as well as those of my guides and using many of the techniques outlined in my book. These are one of a kind, hand made and crafted, wrapped in silver and/or gold-filled wire, or gold upon request, to suit the individuals needs. Universal energy and a lot of love are the main components besides the minerals and crystals.

Ongoing research. I am interested in ongoing research and exploration into the uses of crystals and minerals as our teachers and healers. I also can provide before and after aura photos of healings done with crystals. I plan a future book concerning the energy changes that take place during healings.

You can write to me at: P.O. Box 700830, San Antonio, TX 78270, USA, or email me at: info@wizdombooks.com (make sure you put Wayne on your message).

About the Publisher

Words of Wizdom International, Inc.

For more information about this book, our other products, and how to place an order, you can check the website: www.wizdombooks.com. In North America you can phone 1-800-834-7612 (orders only please).

Other books, divinatory tools and video tapes you can order from Words of Wizdom International, Inc. are:

Teleportation! A Practical Guide
for the Metaphysical Traveler
by Gwen Totterdale, Ph.D.
and Jessica Severn, Ph.D.
Retail Price: $14.95

The Teleportation! Journal
Recording Your Visits to Magical Destinies
by Gwen Totterdale, Ph.D. and Jessica Severn, Ph.D.
Retail Price: $14.95

The Teleportation! Gift Pack Offer:
Teleportation! and The Teleportation! Journal
shrink-wrapped in a gift pack for $24.95

Ceridwen's Handbook of Incense,
Oils and Candles
by Maya Heath
Retail Price: $11.95

Ancient Wizdom Stories
by Dr. Roberta S. Herzog
Retail Price: $12.95

Irish Fairy Cards
by Jaya Moran
(Boxed set of book & 64 cards)
Retail Price: $32.95

Mysteries of Bimini,
When Spirits Come Calling
(Video)
by Adventure Productions
Retail Price: $20.00

Watch for our upcoming titles in 1999-2000 (The New Millenium)

Living the Dolphin Lifestyle
by Gwen Totterdale, Ph.D.

*Planetary Influence*s
by Tracy O'Reilly
and Gwen Totterdale

Irish Alchemy Cards
by Jaya Moran

Kickin' Butts!
by Alan Landers

and much more....!